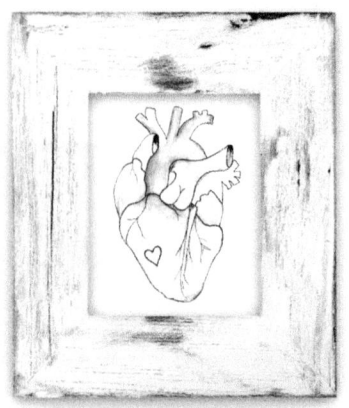

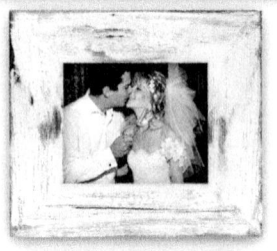

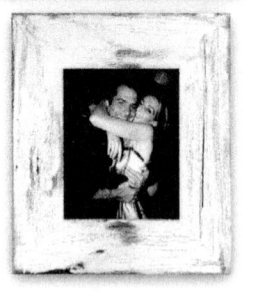

You are here

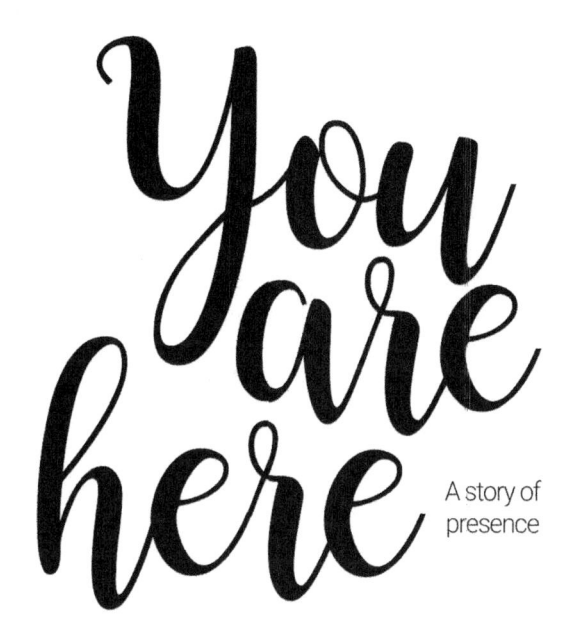

A story of presence

Stefan Brozin
As told to Trevor Waller

by Stefan Brozin,
Sera, Sam, Abby and Ella Brozin
With
Trevor Waller

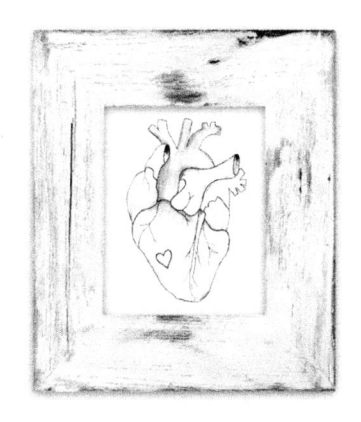

"The point is not what we expect from life,
but rather what life expects of us."

— Viktor Frankl

First published by Stefan Brozin, 2019
Copyright © 2019 by Stefan Brozin

ISBN 978-1-709-06507-1

As told to Trevor Waller
(trevor@tswconsulting.co.za)

Editor: Phillipa Mitchell
(www.phillipamitchell.com)

Heart illustration by Abby Brozin

Cover Design and Typesetting by Gregg Davies
(www.greggdavies.com)

All rights reserved. The moral right of the author has been asserted. No part of this publication may be reproduced, distributed, or transmitted in any form or by any means, including photocopying, recording, or other electronic or mechanical methods, without the prior written permission of the author, except in the case of brief quotations embodied in critical reviews and certain other non-commercial uses permitted by copyright law. Additional copies of this book can be purchased from all leading book retailers worldwide.

"What a caterpillar calls the end of the world,
we call a butterfly."

— Eckhart Tolle

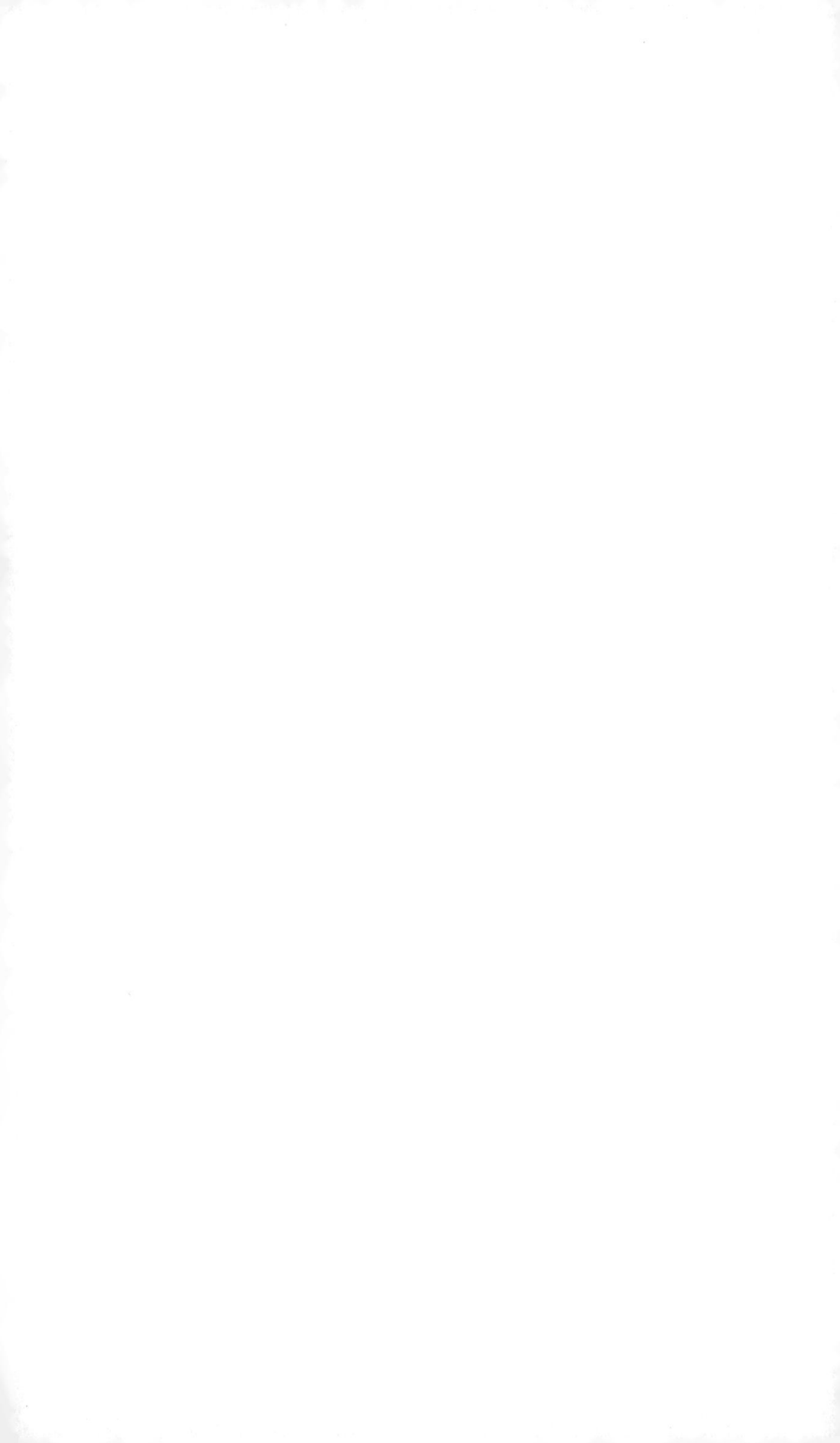

For Jodi, who taught us presence

A NOTE FROM TREVOR WALLER

> "Between stimulus and response there is a space.
> In that space is our power to choose our response.
> In our response lies our growth and our freedom."
>
> — Viktor Frankl

I have known Stefan since grade one. Although we were never good friends and mixed in different circles, Stef was always one of the "good guys". We reconnected at a school reunion, bumping into each other now and again in the months that followed.

I heard, through the Jewish grapevine, that his wife, Jodi, had been diagnosed with cancer. I thought about messaging him but, of course, never got around to it. Next, I heard that Jodi had passed away. This time, I sent Stef a condolence message, offering to support him when he was ready to chat.

I am a Logotherapist which, among other things, means that I am trained to help people to deal with suffering. Logotherapy is the brainchild of Viktor Frankl, the author of the best-selling book "Man's Search for Meaning". The original title of the book was "To Nevertheless Say 'Yes' to Life: A Psychologist Experiences the Concentration Camps".

In the first part of the book, Frankl describes his experiences in the concentration camps during World War Two. Based on these experiences, as well as his observations, Frankl, in the second part of the book, espouses his philosophy, which he calls Logotherapy.

Logos is the Greek word for "meaning". Logo-therapy is, therefore, best described as meaning-based therapy. Frankl disagreed with both Freud—who believed that man is motivated by pleasure—and Adler—who believed that man is motivated by power. In Frankl's view, striving to find meaning in one's life is humankind's primary motivational force. This meaning is unique and specific and must be fulfilled by the individual—and nobody else.

Stef contacted me a few months after Jodi's death. I felt sure that he was contacting me in my capacity as a Logotherapist. I was wrong. He was reaching out to me in my capacity as a ghostwriter. The man, who was sitting opposite me, did not appear to be suffering. To be sure, his grief was palpable. But that was not the overriding emotion that Stef displayed. The man I met that day was strong and positive—

optimistic even. In front of me was living proof of Frankl's beliefs and theories.

The ability to respond to what happens to us in life is what distinguishes man from beast. We may not have a choice over what happens to us—but how we choose to respond is always a choice. Stef and his family had experienced great suffering. Frankl said that suffering, in and of itself, is meaningless. We give it meaning by the way we respond to it. Stef and his children had made a conscious choice to allow their suffering to build them, rather than break them.

Many of the "lessons" in the book are not unique. But that is to miss the point: This is not a theoretical story. This stuff really happened. It is "self-help" in action. It is proof that the "self-helpers" are right: Life is not about what happens to you—it is about what you do with what happens to you.

At first, my logotherapeutic voice was interspersed with Stef's, but that didn't work for me. This is Stef and his children's story. It is *their* voices that must be heard. I offer this note mainly to introduce Frankl, whose quotes and teachings are interspersed throughout the book. But, more than that, I offer it by way of introducing an amazing human being and a beautiful family. There are times when you may feel that Stef's attitude is "too good to be true", but this is not the case—it is both good and it is true. We live in a society where moaning and complaining have become second nature. It does not have to be this way. Stefan and his family show us that humility and gratitude, even in the face of unbearable tragedy, remain a choice.

I am humbled to have worked with Stefan on this book. It is not a story of suffering—it is a story of love, choices and responsibility. It is a story of Logotherapy in action.

I turn again to Frankl to conclude:

> "Everything can be taken from a man but one thing: the last of human freedoms—to choose one's attitude in any given set of circumstances, to choose one's own way."

CONTENTS

Prologue	1
1. Born to be a mother	6
2. Little Me; Big Me	14
3. The meaning of the moment	30
4. Gallery	44
5. Edging God out	60
6. Postscript	70
Reading List	75
Notes	77

It can make us better,
or it can make us bitter.

Ultimately, life is about the choices we make
in the face of what happens to us.

PROLOGUE

> "Death is the crisis of life.
> How a man handles death indicates a
> great deal about how he approaches life."
>
> — Rabbi Maurice Lamm

The week after Jodi's cancer was diagnosed and confirmed was a nightmare. My Little Me raged. "How would I cope? Who would do the admin? How would I look after the kids alone? Should we go overseas to look for a cure? Change her diet? Find a new doctor? Get a second opinion? Perhaps a third?" I vacillated between the proverbial denial and rage. The kids cried. I panicked. Jodi's mom was frantic, while her sister, from her distant home in the USA, went from hopeless to helpless to hysterical in a five-minute telephone conversation.

And then it changed. She changed. I changed. We changed.

After the initial diagnosis, Jodi underwent a six-hour operation at the Milpark Hospital in Johannesburg. While the operation was underway, I took our four children for a walk. It was a perfect summer's day, and we found a small park in the environs of the hospital. Standing shoulder-to-shoulder in a family scrum, we made our choice—we were each going to use this process to find our Big Me. We would not let it break us—we would let it build us.

I looked my children one-by-one in their eyes, and, as the tears welled in my own, I said, "We're going to make the most of this situation. We're going to accept it. We're going to survive it. We will let it teach us. It can make us better, or it can make us bitter. We're going to choose to come out on the other side as better human beings."

And we did.

This book began as the story of the most profound six months of my family's life—the story of how we shepherded Jodi to the next world, how she died with dignity, and how we learned to live, love and laugh amid a terminal illness and an impending farewell. A forever farewell. However, after Jodi's death, my life began to unfold in unexpected ways. The Jo'burg Jewish community is a tight-knit one, and word spread quickly. I found myself being invited to speak to people about our experience. People were surprised at how we, as a family, appeared to be "coping". There was something about the way in which we had not let Jodi's death take us down that resonated with the community—from grief counsellors to school children—and people wanted to know how we had done it. And so, this book transformed from a farewell story into a story of surviving—perhaps even thriving.

The reality is that none of us is immune from suffering. As Viktor Frankl said, *"...to live is to suffer, to survive is to find meaning in the suffering"*.

My family and I found the meaning in our suffering.

I offer this book as a gift to anyone who is suffering as a result of a loved one's suffering. It is important to make this distinction: Jodi was the one who had cancer. She was dying. We bore witness to her suffering, and, although we suffered in turn, we were not the ones facing death. I do not know what it is like to be the actual sufferer.

I am intensely aware that suffering is a deeply personal affair. I am not so arrogant as to believe that

I have words of wisdom for people who have been diagnosed with a terminal illness. What I do know is that, ultimately, life is about the choices we make in the face of what happens to us. We do not choose to suffer. But when suffering hits, in whatever form, we have a choice: to allow it to take us down or to rise up and meet it. My family and I chose to meet it. If the way we did it and the choices we made can bring some form of comfort to anyone who may need it, then this book will have served its purpose.

With love and gratitude,

Stefan, Sera, Sam, Abby and Ella

You can only be where you are.
Fighting it is a waste of time.
You need to embrace it.
You are here, so grab it, be conscious of it
—and give it value.

BORN TO BE A MOTHER

> "Watch any plant or animal and let it teach you
> acceptance of what is, surrender to the Now.
> Let it teach you Being. Let it teach you integrity—
> which means to be one, to be yourself, to be real.
> Let it teach you how to live and how to die, and how not
> to make living and dying into a problem."
>
> — Eckhart Tolle

Jodi was born to be a mother, and our family was her life's work. She took mothering seriously, devoting her life to our children. When, in August 2017, she started running late when it was time to fetch the children from school, forgetting to pay bills and missing appointments, we began to worry.

Abby had been invited to a matric dance and, as always, had turned to her mom to help find her a dress. Jodi was not a relaxed person. Little things made her anxious. Where, under normal circumstances, Jodi would have taken on this task with gusto and habitual anxiety, she was suddenly indifferent. Her lack of concern raised alarm bells. I knew, instinctively, that something was amiss.

After a gastroscopy gave her the all-clear, our GP suggested that a brain scan be conducted. Jodi underwent her scan the day before Rosh Hashanah, the Jewish New Year. After the scan, the doctor asked me to accompany her to her office so that she could show me the scan on her computer.

The walk down the passage was the most intense two minutes of my life. I can remember every moment. Each action I took felt like an eternity. That short walk felt like an hour.

The doctor slipped the disc into her computer and opened the image. A white mass had found its way to the front of my wife's brain. She pointed to it and called it by its name. Jodi had a tumour.

The final results of Jodi's scan were delivered to us on Erev Rosh Hashanah, a time when Jewish families come together to break bread and celebrate life. Rosh Hashanah, which marks the beginning of the Ten Days of Awe, is also known as the Day of Judgement. It is the day when God opens His book, examines one's deeds, and decides who will live, and who will die. The Ten Days conclude with Yom Kippur, the Day of Repentance. It is the day on which one's fate is sealed in the Book of Life and Death. The Ten Days are a time of repentance, prayer and charity. I did not know with any certainty on that day that this was to be Jodi's last Rosh Hashanah but, according to Jewish law, her fate had been sealed the previous Yom Kippur.

People tried to rationalise her acceptance and the grace with which she faced her fate, saying that she exhibited no emotions because the tumour was in her frontal lobe. Or that her executive functioning had diminished. I checked with her doctors and did my own research. It had nothing to do with that. Jodi's attitude towards the tumour was a choice, and her energy and presence became our teachers. We took our lead from her. We could have gone a different route, but when the person who is dying displays no anxiety, who are we to allow our fears and mind-talk to take over?

This is why it is Jodi who is the real hero of this story.

Abby (18) - With struggle comes opportunity

My mom did everything for us—nothing was too much trouble. Even with Sera studying in Cape Town, we would be walking around the shops, and she would see clothes that Sera would like and buy them for her. She covered our books, wrote our speeches, and did our projects.

She wasn't an ordinary mother—she was *extraordinary.* She hardly ever bought anything for herself—everything was always for her kids. When I have children, I want to be just like her.

In a weird way, even though she did everything for us, she also taught us that life is about action. She taught us to make things happen. Since her death, we've realised how much we learned from her. But now we lean on each other and, like her, we do things for each other. She taught us to step up and do what needs doing, whether for yourself or for others.

In the last six months of her life, when she could do little for herself, she taught us a much more important lesson. She taught us to grow up. She taught us to accept life as it is.

Before she started getting sick, my mom had not been happy for a while. Her whole life was about her children. Now, two of her children had left home to study in Cape Town. My younger sister and I were relying less on her and becoming more independent. She hadn't worked in a long time, and wasn't sure what she was going to do with her life. I remember my dad telling her that she should get a job. She spent a lot of time playing Sudoku on her phone, almost as if she was bored with life.

This may sound weird, but, when she got sick, she stopped being anxious. In those last six months of her life, she was completely content. She was strong, and she was wise. She was happier than she had ever been. She did not fight what was happening to her. She did everything the doctors told her to do. The cancer was bigger than her, and so she had to accept that fighting against it was not going to make any difference.

She used her last six months to take in and appreciate the love that everyone was giving her. She knew what was going on, and she chose to use the opportunity to appreciate the time that she had left. She smiled all the time —much more than before.

Before she got sick, my mom used to worry about trivial things. Her illness helped her focus on what was important, and we actually watched her anxiety reduce. It was amazing to see how she transformed. She totally embraced what was happening her. She was just happy where she was. She never complained. And she definitely didn't lose her sense of humour. I remember when the new Checkers opened at BluBird, and someone said she should go with them to see it, she said, "I'd rather go to treatment than go to the shops!"

I learned in Jewish Studies that you leave the world when you have fulfilled your purpose. My mom's purpose in life was to raise her children. And she did. I really believe that she had fulfilled her purpose. She did not fight death. And her acceptance helped us to accept her death.

When my dad told us that he wanted to write a book about our experience, I came up with the title. It is what we learned from our mom. You can only be where you are. Fighting it is a waste of time. You need to embrace it. *You are here*, so grab it, be conscious of it, and give it value.

Yesterday, when I was coming home on the bus, I found myself looking out of the window and noticing how beautiful everything was. I appreciated the jacaranda trees and the joggers and the dog walkers. In the past, I would have just been on my phone. I noticed the sky and the clouds, and I was grateful for them. Now, I never leave home without kissing my dad goodbye. My mom's death taught me presence and gratitude for what is. I am here.

Big Me lives here, in the now, conscious and present to the moment, in full acceptance of what is. Big Me does not defend, he does not judge, and he does not resist.

Ultimately, Little Me and Big Me cannot coexist—You are either giving your power to Little Me or you are taking back your power by consciously tuning into Big Me thoughts.

2

LITTLE ME; BIG ME

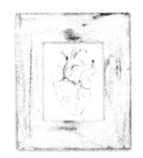

> "Always say 'yes' to the present moment. What could be more futile, more insane, than to create inner resistance to what already is? What could be more insane than to oppose life itself, which is now and always now? Surrender to what is. Say 'yes' to life—and see how life suddenly starts working for you rather than against you."
>
> — Eckhart Tolle

*J*odi's diagnosis was not my first experience of cancer. My father died when I was seven years old—from a brain tumour. Now, here I was, a forty-nine-year-old man, about to lose my wife to the same disease that had not only killed my father but inexorably changed my life. When Jodi was diagnosed, I did not know that I would be burying her the day before my fiftieth birthday. What I did know, with absolute certainty, was that my life had prepared me for this, and that, in a strange and inexplicable way, I had been preparing my children for it too.

When you are seven years old and your dad dies, you learn, without being able to put words to it, that life is fragile and fleeting. I did not know it at the time, but, when my dad passed away, a seed was planted. As a little boy, I knew that moments are impermanent, and that, because they are impermanent, they must be valued.

Years later, I would give my inner child a name: I called him my Little Me—which he was, quite literally. But Little Me is not a child, just as Big Me is not an adult: Little Me and Big Me are states of being.

When you are a child, you do not know that you are *not* the voice in your head. As a child, you *are* your thoughts. These thoughts are all you know, they are frightening and disturbing—and you literally become them. Many of us grow from frightened, disturbed children into frightened and disturbed adults, unable to distinguish between ourselves and the voice in our head.

Adults, for the most part, have more sophisticated coping mechanisms than children and are better able to masquerade as competent. Despite the adult veneer, however, Little Me continues to shout loudly inside their heads.

As I grew older, Little Me constantly worried, obsessed about other people and what they thought of him, becoming agitated at the slightest unexpected occurrence, trying to control the outcome of every event. Little Me missed the moments, asked "why?" and, unable to find the answer, became more obsessive, more controlling, and more fearful. I read books, I studied with Rabbis, and I searched for meaning. Nothing quite hit the mark. And then, one day, as I was browsing the bookshelves in a local bookshop, I found the book that would change my life.

The Power of Now.

I had never heard of Eckhart Tolle, but the title of his book hit a spot somewhere deep inside me. My hand reached for it, its name echoing in my mind.

The power of now…"What is that? What does it mean?"

It is a small book. I turned it over and read the blurb. I knew that I had to read it. And so began the longest read of my life. I spent almost a year reading its one-hundred-and-ninety pages. It became my bible—my daily scripture. With a pencil and highlighter in my hand, I read two or three pages a day, making notes, highlighting lines and re-reading them.

The Power of Now allowed me to heal my past and correct my present. It also unwittingly prepared me for my future.

It is as it is…

The present moment is sometimes unacceptable, unpleasant, or awful. It is as it is. Observe how the mind labels it and how this labelling process, this continuous sitting in judgment, creates pain and unhappiness. By watching the mechanics of the mind, you step out of its resistance patterns, and you can then allow the present moment to be. This will give you a taste of the state of inner freedom from external conditions, the state of true inner peace. Then see what happens and take action if necessary or possible.

Accept—then act. *Whatever the present moment contains, accept it as if you had chosen it.* Always work with it, not against it. Make it your

> friend and ally, not your enemy. This will miraculously transform your whole life.[1]

The Power of Now, p.29

In the months that I spent poring over the book, glimpses of *presence* began revealing themselves to me. At first, they were mere moments where I found myself not in my head, but rather present in the moment—not judging, just observing. Meditating without meditating. Not reliving a past experience or anticipating a future event. Just here. Now. Because Big Me lives here, in the now, conscious and present to the moment, in full acceptance of what is. Big Me does not defend, he does not judge, and he does not resist.

Shortly after I finished reading the book, I was having my weekly breakfast catch-up with my mom when I received a phone call. Ella, our youngest daughter, who had been born with a heart condition, had suddenly stopped breathing. I abandoned my Macon and eggs and rushed to the hospital. Presence was the furthest thing from my mind. All I was thinking was, "What if I arrive at the hospital to find that she's dead?"

I raced through the hospital, down the stairs to the Casualty ward—and there she was, lying in bed, bawling her eyes out. Never before have I been so grateful for a crying child. It had been a false alarm, and Ella was fine. I spent some time comforting her, and then, reassured by the doctors that she would be all right, I left the hospital, grateful and relieved.

When I arrived home, I realised how hungry I was, having not finished my breakfast. I filled a bowl with cereal, covered it with ice-cold milk, and sat down on my patio to eat it. As I lifted the spoon, not only did I feel it in my hand, I *noticed* it. A sparkle of sunshine reflected off its shiny surface. I breathed in deeply and smelt the cereal. I noticed each individual grain. I felt the mixture of milk and grains in my mouth. I allowed myself to taste the cereal. I chewed purposefully. I swallowed carefully. I have never eaten a bowl of cereal more slowly. Each mouthful was a sensory delight. I paused between each spoonful, noticing my pool, my garden, and my dogs. I was as grateful for a breathing daughter as I was for that bowl of cereal. Both were gifts that I had previously taken for granted.

It was then that a light went on in my head, and I understood the meaning of the *power of now*. I grasped the blessing of the present moment. Presence is not an intellectual thing. It is not something we think about. It is something we *allow* ourselves to experience. When you bring all your senses to the present moment and accept that it is as it is, whether you want it to be or not, when you are grounded in the moment, neither reminiscing nor anticipating, just experiencing, that is when you are present. You are here.

I have spent my life running from tumours. Tumours take fathers away, leaving little boys alone and fearful. My Little Me saw tumours in every unexpected life event. I spent years in therapy trying to understand that *not* everything is a tumour, that another catastrophe is *not* always around the corner. But, lo and behold, here was a real-life tumour. It was back. It was big. And it was sitting on Jodi's brain.

After Jodi's diagnosis, the Rosh Hashanah meal at my sister's house was subdued and solemn. The realisation that our lives had changed forever hit each of us at different moments. There was one moment that I remember in particular, where part of the meal involved dipping an apple in honey and asking God "to renew us for a good and sweet new year". The irony of the moment was not lost on any of us. I tried in vain to stay present, but my Little Me was having none of it.

I barely slept that night. Thoughts raced through my mind. I relived my childhood. I wondered how I would manage and how the children would cope. My son was in matric, my daughter at university in Cape Town. Both were about to write their final exams.

I told myself I would never be happy again.

For the three days following Jodi's diagnosis, Little Me's voice dominated. Every now and then, I would catch a glimpse of Big Me. Each time I did, I allowed his voice to comfort me.

"This is where you are. Be here now, and deal with what is," Big Me would say.

I endeavoured to stay present. I knew that I was no longer that helpless seven-year-old boy—I was a father, a husband, and an adult with resources.

We were told that Dr Zorio at the Milpark Hospital was the best doctor for us to see, so Jodi was transferred. People had advised me to keep the details from the children—that somehow, their *not* knowing would be easier than arming them with information and facts. I knew differently—having been spared the reality of my father's tumour, I knew that there is no such thing as too much information. Not knowing allows the imagination to run rampant —and it does not run to good places. I knew, from the outset, that this was going be a family journey. Although we had spent our lives on family holidays, this was not a trip we had planned, and it was certainly not going to be a holiday. But, we would be taking this journey together, of that I was certain. And so, that day at Milpark hospital, the whole family was there, staring at the tumour on Dr Zorio's computer screen.

Dr Zorio dispensed medication to bring down the swelling on Jodi's brain and confirmed that her operation would take place three days later. We left the hospital. Jodi displayed no anxiety at all. For someone who had been so anxious for most of her life, seeing her so calm was almost unsettling. What was happening, however, was that Jodi had taken the lead. And, despite our obvious fear, we began to follow her example.

We went to *Koi*, one of Jodi's favourite restaurants, the night before the operation. Dinner was good, and, in between the tears, we laughed and allowed ourselves to enjoy the evening. A couple, whom we know, and who knew about the impending operation, expressed disbelief that we were out enjoying ourselves. This was to be the first of many such encounters. It was almost as if people wanted—or even *needed*—us to be dramatic, depressed, and freaked out. The thing is, we *were* sad, and we *were* scared, but we knew that creating drama around our shared reality was not going to help us. As far as we were concerned, the future remained unknown, and there was no point in going there.

Walking back to the car later that evening, Jodi, who was struggling to balance, cracked a joke, and we all laughed. To the casual observer, we were a family whose mother was slightly drunk. Despite an impending operation on her brain, she chose laughter—and we did too. Jodi's sense of humour carried us, and her, right through to the very end.

The next day, while she was in theatre, we had our family scrum in the hospital garden. This was the moment when I put my Little Me to rest and allowed my Big Me to take control. Looking back, it was also the moment that each of my children gave *their* Big Me's permission to emerge. We were becoming a family of Big Me's.

After my father died, I became completely obsessed with thoughts of "Am I alone?"; "Who's going to look after me?"; "What will happen a moment from now?"; "What will happen tomorrow?"; "Why did this happen?". I became my thoughts. I was my thoughts—I was a lost, frightened little boy. Little Me was little me. He controlled me and created my experiences.

But then, it dawned on me—Big Me could choose his thoughts too. It took years of searching, therapy and, finally, *The Power of Now*, for me to understand that Little Me was born as a result of my experiences, but that he was not me. I did not need to allow Little Me to control me. I did not have to hold onto fear or guilt. I did not need to see every swerve as a potential tumour.

The realisation that I could observe my thoughts—that I could have different Big Me thoughts—liberated me. I gave myself permission to become an adult when I consciously and deliberately turned down the volume on Little Me and tuned purposefully into the voice of my Big Me.

When you allow Big Me to take charge, you become an observer of your thoughts. This is the first step towards acceptance and presence. Little Me struggles to accept things as they are. He wants people to behave in a certain way, and he wants life to work out *his* way. He wants perfection. Big Me knows that life is perfect as it is, no matter how difficult it is. Ultimately, Little Me and Big Me cannot coexist—You are either giving your power to Little Me, or you are taking back your power by consciously tuning into Big Me thoughts.

On that day, when that real-life tumour eventually did present itself, I gave Big Me the opportunity to handle the tumour. Big Me's first job was to comfort my Little Me. I began to consciously and deliberately nurture my Little Me. I told him that he was not responsible for everything that happened in the world. I noted his fear, anxiety and guilt, but I did not take on these feelings. I became an observer of my Little Me thoughts, instead of being them.

Sera (22) - I am not my thoughts

My dad is the calmest, most laid-back person you will ever meet. From the outside, it is easy to judge him and believe that he is in denial. How can you lose your partner of thirty-five years and still be okay? What is he hiding? What's wrong with him? Is he repressing his feelings? The truth is that the only thing that my dad is *not* doing is being dramatic. He thinks deeply, and he feels intensely. What my dad knows, and what he taught me is that he is *not* his thoughts, and he is *not* his feelings.

While my mom was sick, my dad gave me a book called *The Untethered Soul: The Journey Beyond Yourself* to read. I finally understood what he had been trying to explain to me for all these years.

In the book, the author, Michael A Singer, says:

"There is nothing more important to true growth than realizing that you are not the voice of the mind—you are the one who hears it."[2]

After reading the book, I could be with my mom and have all sorts of thoughts—sadness, fear, guilt, worry—and still enjoy the moment, because I am not my thoughts. I can acknowledge my thoughts, but I do not need to become them. It is a strange concept, but it allowed me to enjoy all the moments.

Our family's blessing is that we had six months to say goodbye to Mom. We had time to make sure that we would have no regrets.

We were able to tell her that we loved her, to say sorry for some of the things that we had done, to hold her, and to love her.

Like my mom, I also used to be an anxious person. I used to worry about all sorts of stupid things, especially material things—such as what I was wearing. Before my mom fell ill, I wouldn't say that we were the perfect family, but nothing ever really went wrong for us. We used to go on holidays together, and our parents rarely fought. Before my mom was diagnosed, I truly believed that these kinds of things happened to other families. In those six months, I learned that life is short and that anything can happen to you.

I remember one day when she was lying in her bed, and I went to lie down next to her. I've never felt so present, so *in the moment*. It was pouring with rain outside, and I was holding her hand. It was probably one of the best moments of my life. I did not allow my thoughts to take me away from the moment. There was no worrying about stuff that didn't matter, and I refused to allow myself to have any thoughts about the future. I remember holding her hand tightly. I lay with her, and I fell asleep. I'll never forget that.

Before she got sick, Mom often complained that nobody appreciated her and that no one showed her love. During those six months, we showered her with love and appreciation. Sometimes, she would say, "It's enough!" because we wouldn't stop telling her how much we loved her. But we didn't stop. We didn't let our Little Me thoughts get in the way of loving her while we still could.

No matter what is happening to you, you can choose to enjoy the moment for what it is.

Acceptance of the present must learn to cohabit with the human capacity for hope.

Outcomes are for the future; experiences are for the present.

THE MEANING OF THE MOMENT

"The meaning of life differs from man to man, from day to day, from hour to hour. What matters, therefore, is not the meaning of life in general but rather the specific meaning of a person's life at a given moment ... Therein he cannot be replaced, nor can his life be repeated."

— Viktor Frankl

*I*t is not easy to become an observer of your thoughts. When you realise that you are not your thoughts, you become present and engaged, and you learn to welcome what *is*. Ultimately, this is what Jodi taught us. She never allowed herself to entertain thoughts of the future. She never asked, "What if the treatment doesn't work?", or "What will happen to the kids?", or "Who will look after my dogs?". She did not allow her mind-talk to slip into the future—she stayed in the here and now. The energy of her present-moment awareness buoyed us, forcing us to stay with her in the here and now too. We stopped listening to our Little Me voices and enjoyed every moment we had with her. We learned that no matter what is happening to you, you can choose to enjoy the moment for what it is.

People thought we were mad. "How can you enjoy chemo?" they asked. But we really did—because Jodi's chemotherapy sessions gave us precious, uninterrupted time with her. When friends asked me how I was coping, I always replied quite simply: "I don't think about it!" When I walked down the hospital passage, I brought all my awareness to that moment. I noticed the walls, the signs, and the people. I put one foot in front of the other, and I gave thanks for legs that could carry me unaided. I would bring myself to where I was, instead of going into the future. That is where my growth lay.

Every time I caught myself going down Little Me's future-tunnel of fear and anxiety, I would immediately bring myself back to my present—to what *is*. I would hold Jodi's hand, see her, notice her, and listen to her talking. I relished the experience for everything it was, not for what could be, and not for what would be—just for what it was. All I could think was, "She is here. I am here. That is what matters. This is the *only* thing that matters."

Sadly, while Jodi's operation succeeded in removing the tumour, it did not eradicate the cancer. Dr Zorio confirmed that she had what is known as a Glioblastoma (GBM) tumour. The prognosis was clear. The best-case scenario was a year. The reality was half that.

After the first operation, and despite his attempts to be positive, I could tell by Dr Zorio's face that he was not overly optimistic. I did some of my own research on GBM tumours and, despite the miracle case of someone who had lived for twenty years with it, deep down I knew that time was short and that we would have to embrace every precious second we had with Jodi.

Nonetheless, the end was still a while off, and so began the arduous journey of chemoradiation—a combination of chemotherapy and radiation treatments. The doctors proposed thirty-three radiation treatments, five days on and two days off, combined with oral chemotherapy treatment. Jodi's friends took it upon themselves to organise a schedule of family and friends who would take it in turns to accompany her to her radiation treatments. From the outset, there was an almost silent acknowledgement that this would be a special time to be with Jodi. Deep down, I believe people realised that as difficult as the experience might be, it would also be life-changing. In the end, we were quite literally turning people away because there were more people than there were treatments.

The doctors planned on starting the radiation two weeks after the operation. When I looked at the dates, I realised that they clashed with a planned family holiday in Zanzibar. I discussed this with the medical team, and they brought the treatment dates forward. All things being equal, we would go on our family holiday together. Hope truly does spring eternal. Giving up was not an option. Acceptance of the present must learn to cohabit with the human capacity for hope.

I cherished those drives with Jodi to her radiation sessions. On our drives to the hospital, she smiled and never complained. When we arrived, she would greet everyone, never failing to express gratitude to each person who helped her—not just the doctors, but all the 'little people'—the receptionist, the helpers and the nurses, all of whose names she knew. I saw a similar phenomenon when my mom suffered a stroke a few years back.

When it happens, and if they allow it, a catastrophe has the power to fill the sufferer with a newfound sense of gratitude. A sense of humility creeps in, together with an incredible awareness and appreciation for everything. This certainly came over Jodi. It was during this time of witnessing Jodi's appreciation for all the people who were assisting her that I allowed myself to become present and be grateful too. I began to say to myself, "This is all there is—this is the experience. Don't worry about the outcome."

Being unattached to the outcome is a crucial component of Big Me thinking. Little Me is obsessed with results and outcomes—but outcomes are for the future. Experiences are for the present. Of course, the doubts and the fears crept in—I am not superhuman—but I gave them as little airtime as possible. As a family, we found a way to embrace the experience and enjoy our moments with Jodi. And while we did, we witnessed a new Jodi emerging—a Jodi who was calm and all-embracing—and we were led by her example.

Jodi became obsessed with food—cheese in particular. Despite the best efforts of her friends to keep her away from sugar and carbs, Jodi was having none of it. She was obsessed with hospital tramezzini, and would often make us pop into the Linksfield Clinic, whose tramezzini she declared to be the best in Johannesburg. Her newfound enthusiasm for food matched her newfound enthusiasm for life. It was infectious, and we allowed ourselves to be infected too.

With the end of the thirty-three treatments fast approaching, we asked our doctors if we could go to Zanzibar. Our GP, the chemo doctor, as well as the radiation doctor, all said that we could go. The only person left to consult was the oncologist, Dr Rapoport. We chatted to him the day before we were scheduled to leave, but he was not in favour of Jodi leaving South Africa. He warned of all sorts of possible complications if she accompanied us. Ultimately, the decision was ours, but he was exceptionally concerned about the risk of being stuck in Zanzibar with a critically-ill patient.

We returned home that day and found ourselves gathered together for yet another family meeting on our patio. We vacillated, in an open and heartfelt way, between "If Mommy's not coming, we're not going either" to "We've just finished exams—we all need the break", and every other argument of pros and cons under the sun. Eventually, we made a decision. I would take the kids to Zanzibar and Jodi's mom would stay with her. The minute the decision was made, I found myself rushing to the police station to get an affidavit giving me permission to travel as a single parent with my children.

The first few hours in Zanzibar were difficult. I checked my phone often, and if I had not heard from Jodi or her mom for a few hours, my thoughts began to race. Eventually, her mom *did* call—Jodi had suffered a seizure. It was her first seizure since being diagnosed, and we were two-thousand-five-hundred kilometres away when it happened. She had been rushed to the Linksfield clinic and, although she was still sedated, she appeared to be fine.

Having just decided to come to Zanzibar, we were now faced with another dilemma—do we go home?

The following day, Jodi had regained consciousness, and we could speak to her. It was Monday, and the next flight out of Zanzibar was only that Thursday. We were planning to be there until the following Monday. When we told Jodi that we were considering taking the Thursday flight, she was having none of it. "Stay in Zanzibar for the week," she said, "And, more importantly, have a good time!"

Zanzibar is so beautiful, but how does one give oneself permission to enjoy the beauty in the midst of such a nightmare? We found a way—we made a family decision that we would have a good holiday, no matter what. We would do it because we needed it and because Jodi wanted us to be there. And we did. We swam, we snorkelled, we ate good food, and we relaxed on the beach. We had a good break. There were, of course, moments of anxiety, but we acknowledged them and allowed ourselves to be both happy and anxious.

The reality was that there was nothing we could do for Jodi, whether we were there or not. We had a choice—be depressed and go home, or embrace where we are and enjoy what *is*. I was in a beautiful place, the sun was shining, and I was with my four beautiful children. I chose to have a fantastic time.

Again, we were confronted with disbelief by acquaintances who were holidaying at the same time as us. But, it wasn't about them, it was about us—we had chosen to be in the moment, and the moment was good for us. At the same time, Jodi and her mom were getting to spend a week together, just the two of them. We were right to be in Zanzibar, and it was right for Jodi and her mom to have their time together. As much as we missed Jodi and worried about her, she and her mom were spending their last days together. Our being miserable in the midst of the beauty that is Zanzibar would not have served anyone.

The truth is that life unfolds the way it is meant to—and there is always choice.

Upon our return, we had yet another decision to make. We had planned to spend two weeks in Cape Town after Zanzibar. All the arrangements had been made. We decided that the children would go to Cape Town, and I would stay home with Jodi.

The children had a fantastic holiday in Cape Town. They looked after each other and got to be responsible for themselves. Without adults around, and despite the trauma that each of them was coping with, they not only had a bonding experience second to none, but they also had time to be there for each other. During their stay in Cape Town, they each discovered their Big Me selves. It was to be a seminal holiday for all of them.

There is a quiet that descends over Jo'burg in December that can only be described as sublime. During that time, Jodi and I spent two beautiful weeks together. We were alone, at home, with no children and no staff. We lived from moment to moment. Each morning we would decide what we were going to eat, and then we would walk slowly through the supermarket together, carefully choosing the perfect loaf of bread, and then its filling, deliberating over how we would prepare our sandwiches. After hours of careful preparation, we would sit down together to eat, savouring each precious mouthful. We went out for ice cream together—it had never tasted more delicious or enjoyable.

We had each other, and we had the now—what more could we ask for? Our cup ran over for two blissful weeks. When our time with those we love is limited, slowing down to enjoy the bounty of its gifts is so effortless.

Sam (20) - It's not a dying story—it's a living story

I wasn't always a nice brother. I used to fight with my sisters about such trivial things. I remember getting so irritated waiting for my older sister to get ready. Now I don't scream at her. Those things, the *little* things, don't matter anymore.

My mom's diagnosis and the six months we spent with her made me a better person—and

I thank God for blessing with me with such a wonderful opportunity. There was a great lesson in this experience—we need to learn to take each moment seriously. None of us knows how much time we have, yet we walk around with the illusion that we have forever. We don't. We wait until we know that we have six months to live, and then suddenly we value the important things in life. The challenge is to value our lives *now*. We shouldn't wait to be diagnosed with a terminal illness before we start valuing our lives and appreciating the moments.

The funny thing is that, for as long as I can remember, I had a feeling that my mom would die of cancer. I always had a suspicion that she would die before my dad. This was unnerving, and I developed some unusual OCD habits to counterbalance my fears. For instance, I would touch things four times, or close and open taps, believing, in a weird way, that I if I did these things, nobody would die. When my mom was diagnosed with cancer, I realised that my OCD habits couldn't prevent bad things from happening. I no longer do those things, choosing instead to focus on the things that *really* matter—the people I love.

My mom used to hate it when I fought with my sisters. When she fell ill, I stopped. She wanted us to make an effort to appreciate each other. In the last six months of my mom's life, my Big Me emerged, and I finally grew up.

The turning point for me was when my dad invited Cameron Hogg from Hospice to come to the house to talk to us. He said that a good mother never gives a child something that is not good for them. "Your mother is giving you an amazing gift," he said, "She's mothered you sufficiently, and now she's going to teach you something else—something really valuable." That gift, according to Cameron, was the gift of consciousness. This must be the most valuable gift that any parent can give their child.

"When you are conscious, you realise that life is short and that you have to value each and every moment," Cameron continued, "Your heart is going to break, but you're going to build it back double the size. You're going to have more compassion, and you're going to see life differently to people your age. This is the blessing and the gift that your mother is giving you."

After Cameron's visit, I became a different person. I was writing my final matric exams when my mom was diagnosed, and yet I found a way to cope. I had always wanted to study in Cape Town, but I needed a good matric to get in. This was important to my mom too. I found a way to be with my mom and my sisters in a loving and grateful way while focussing on my studies. In the past, I would have been the biggest grouch. But things were different now—I *had* to study, my mom was dying, and our house was always full of people. I didn't get irritated, nor did I take my frustrations out on other people.

Even though my mom is no longer here, I can feel her everywhere. I'm coping so much better than I thought I would. As a family, those six months with mom gave us closure. We got to say everything we wanted to say. I have no feelings of guilt or regret. I got to apologise for my bad behaviour in the past and to make peace with my mom.

Life without her is our "new normal".

Everyone dies. I had nineteen years with her. That is how it was meant to be. Life goes on. Mom's death was a lesson for us. It brought us closer, it showed us to love each other more, and it taught us not to be afraid.

The last thing my mom said to me before she slipped away was, "I love you". I will treasure those words and that moment for as long as I live.

4

GALLERY

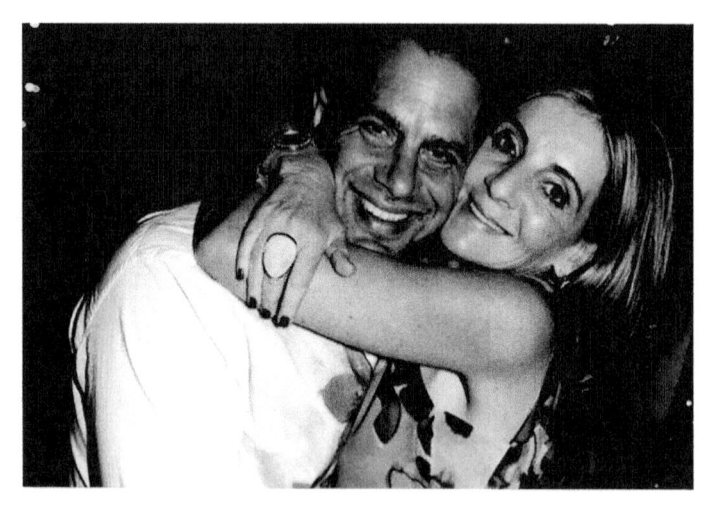

Stefan & Jodi at Ella's Bat Mitzvah

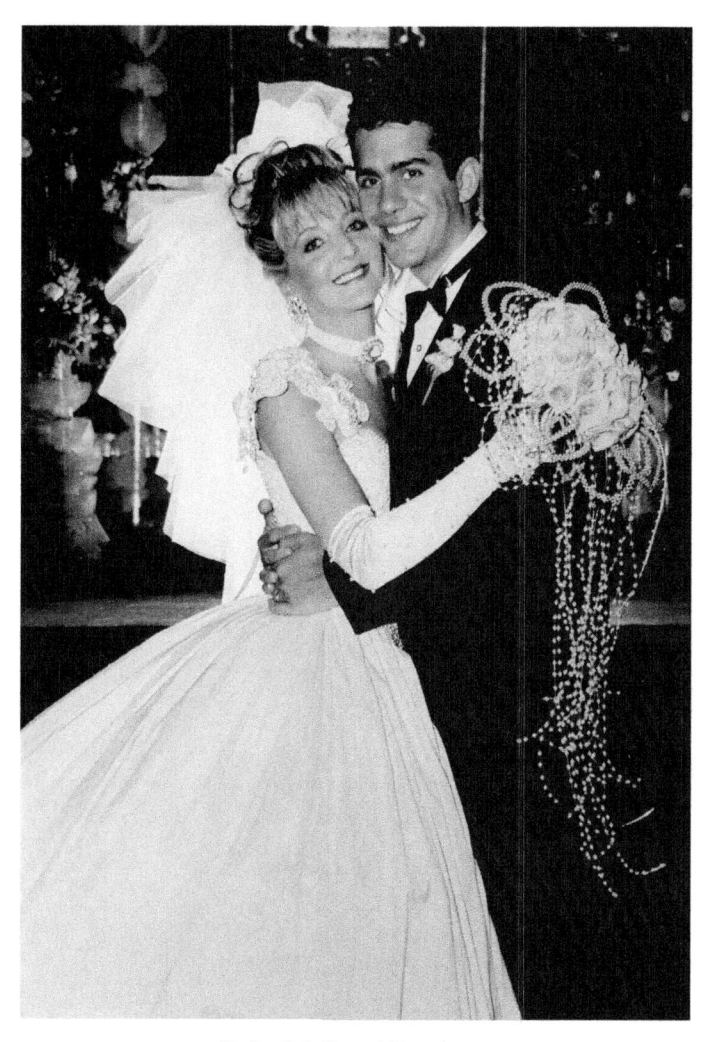

Stefan & Jodi: wedding picture

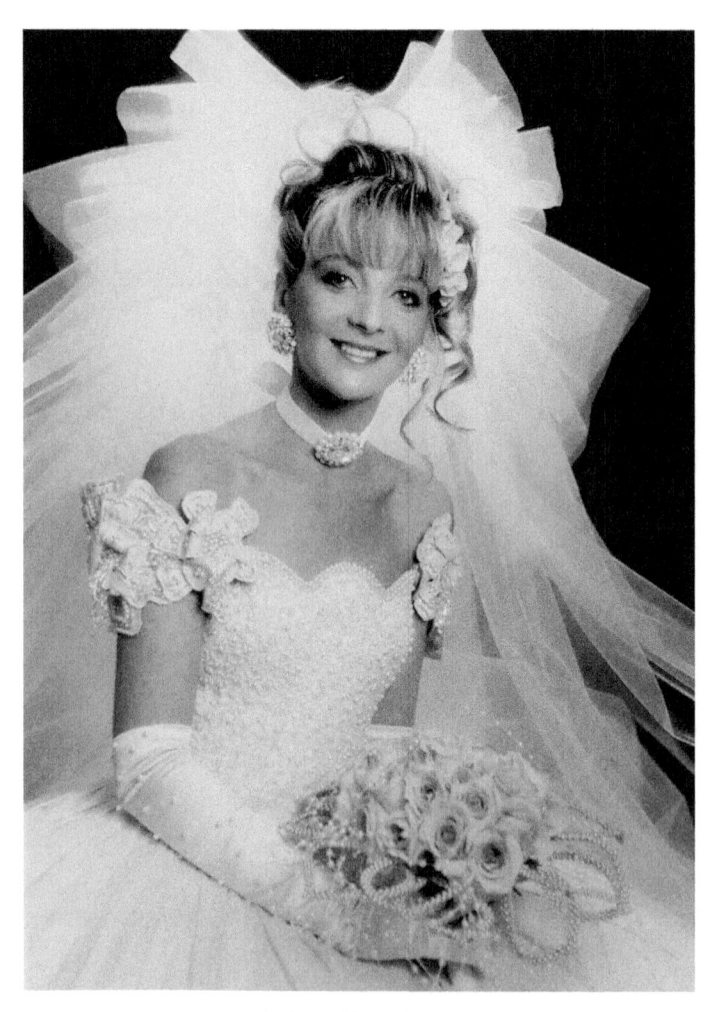

Jodi: wedding picture

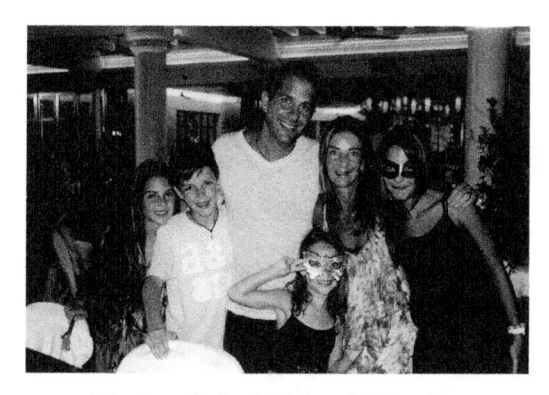

Abby, Sam, Stefan, Jodi, Sera & Ella at New Year's Eve party in Phuket, Thailand

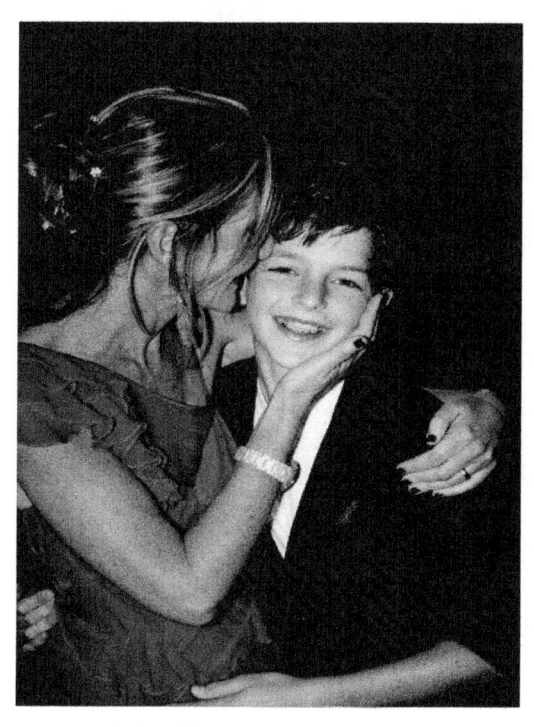

Jodi and Sam at Sam's Bar Mitzvah

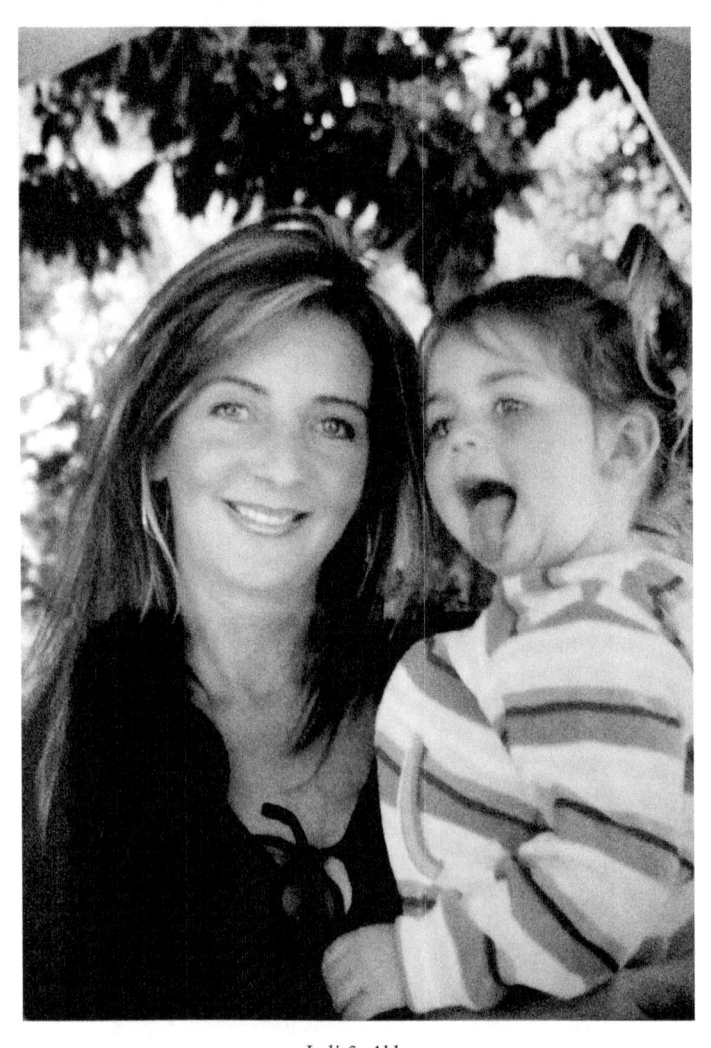

Jodi & Abby

GALLERY | 49

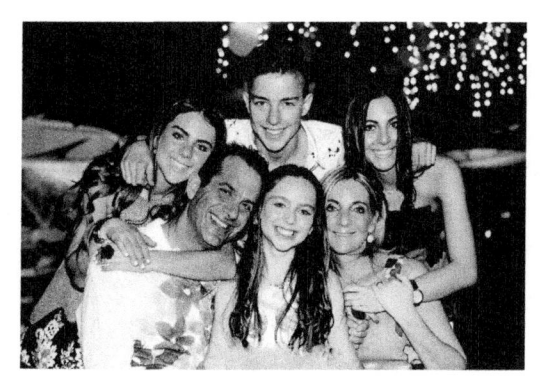

Family at Ella's Bat Mitzvah party

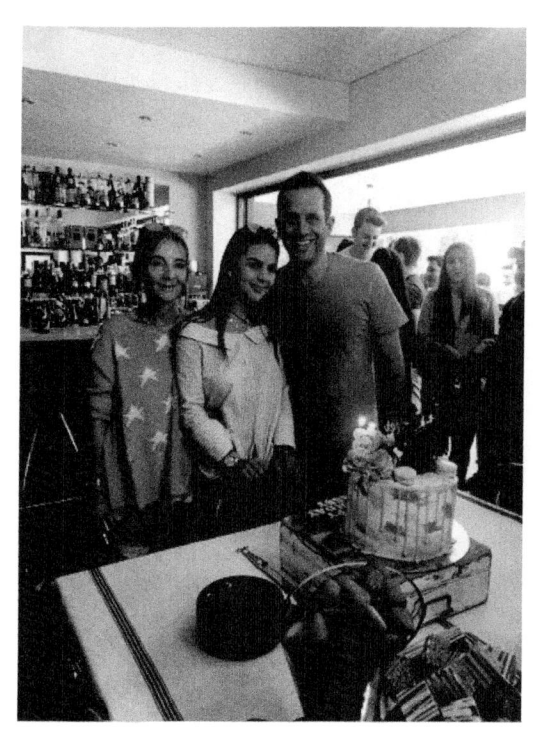

Jodi, Abby and Stefan at Abby's 16th birthday

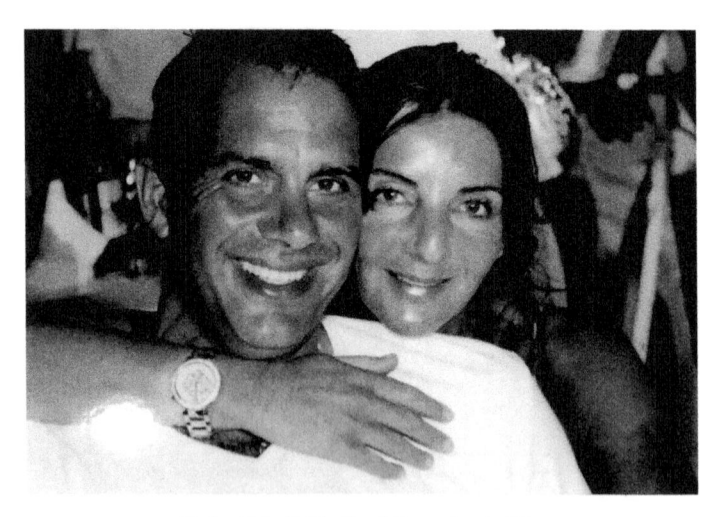

Stefan & Jodi, Thailand December holiday

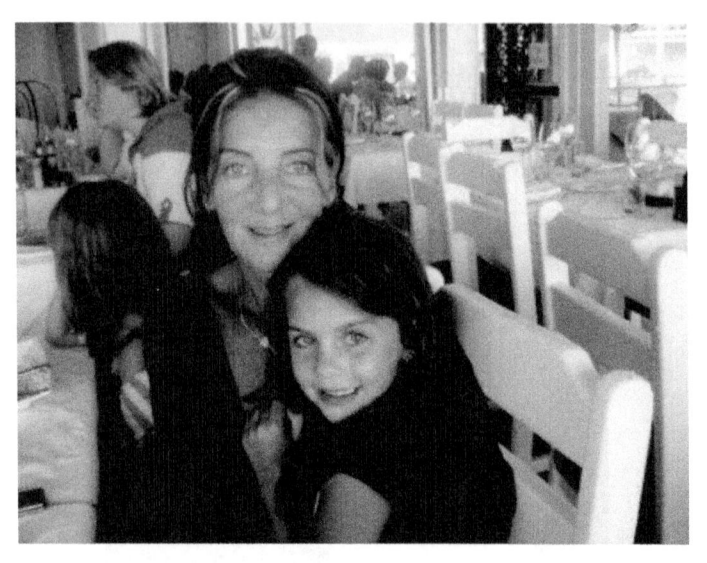

Jodi and Abby

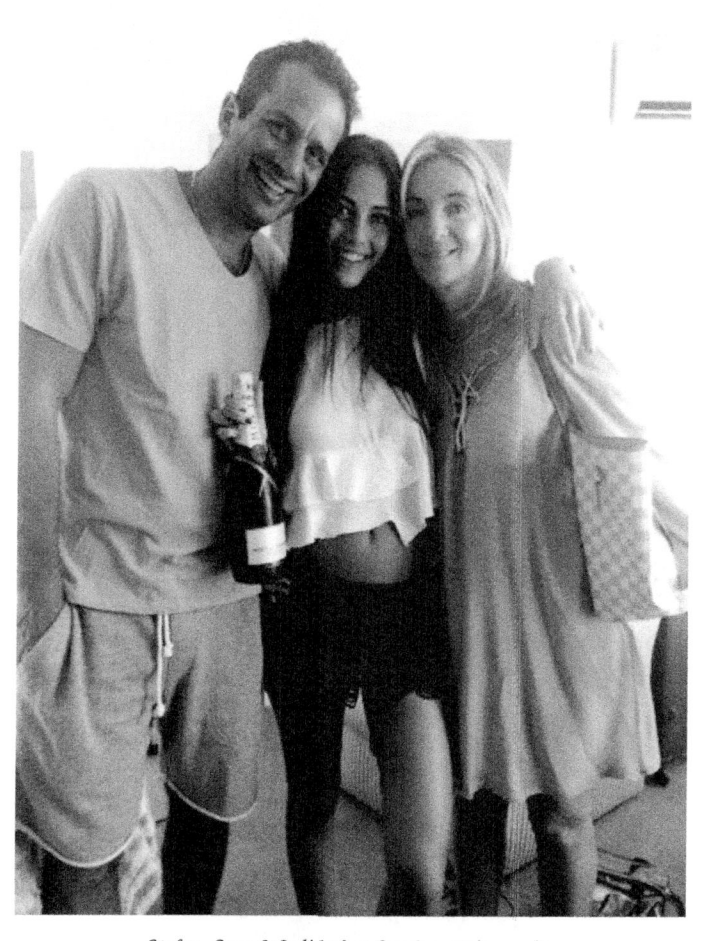

Stefan, Sera & Jodi before Sera's matric results

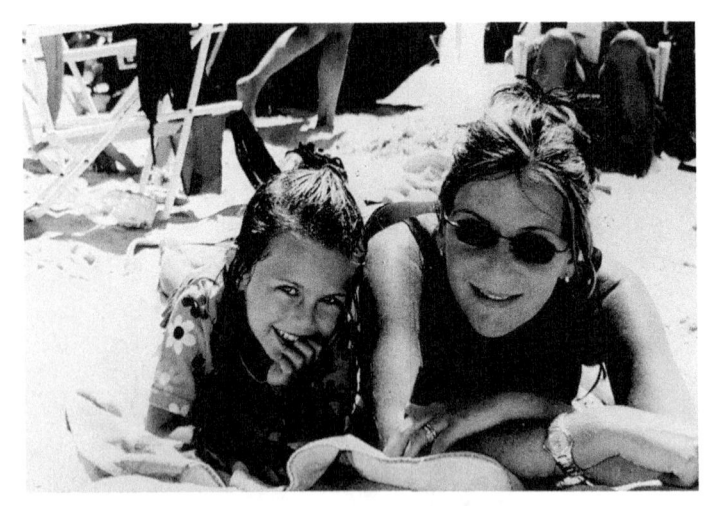

Jodi & Sera in Plettenberg Bay, December holiday

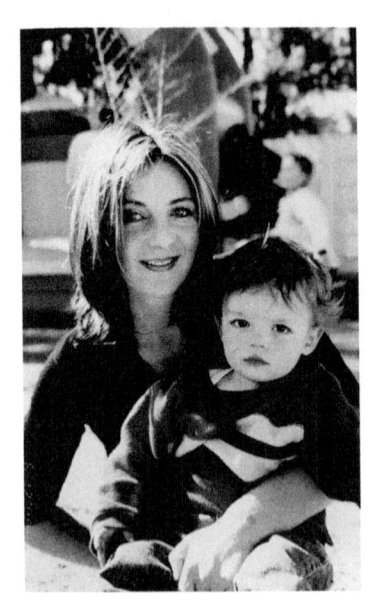

Jodi and Sam at birthday party

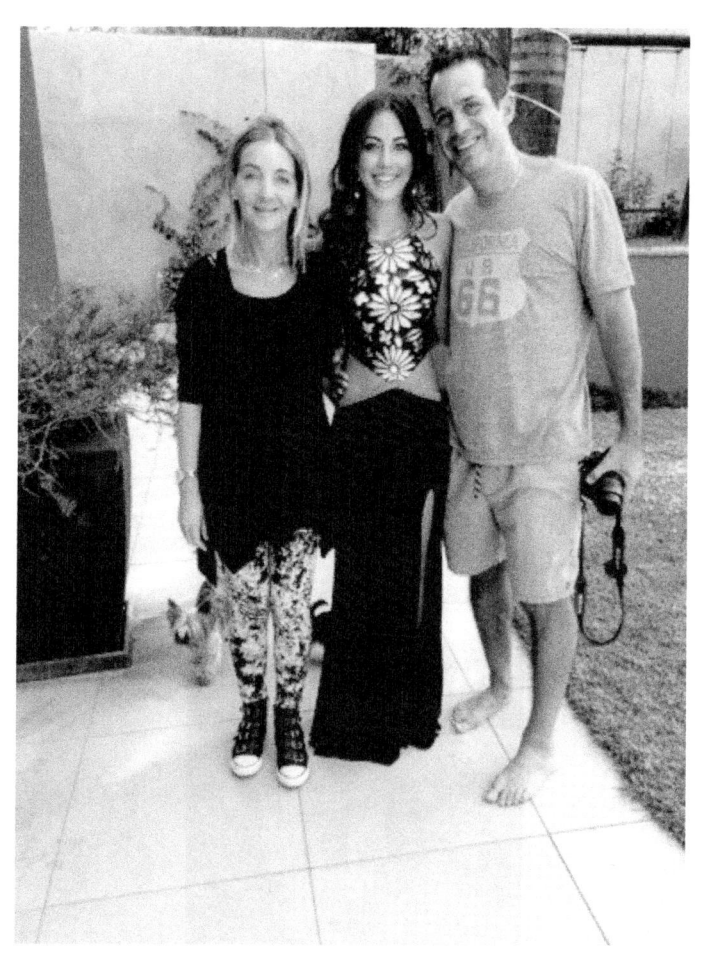

Jodi, Sera & Stefan at Sera's matric dance

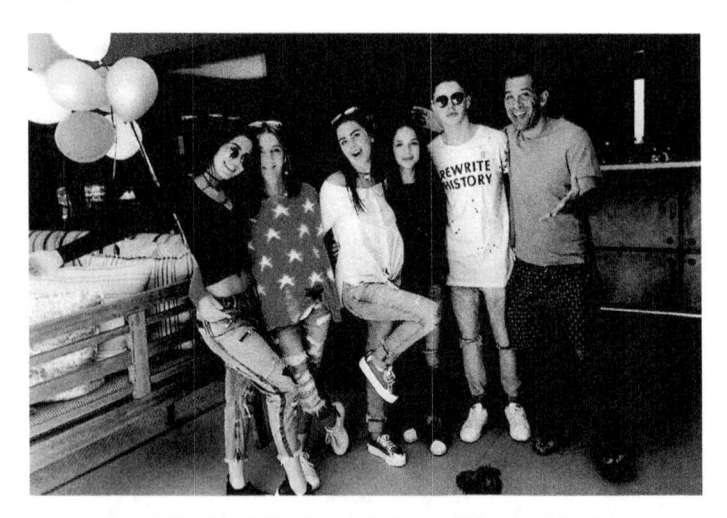

Sera, Jodi, Abby, Ella, Sam & Stefan at Abby's 16th birthday party

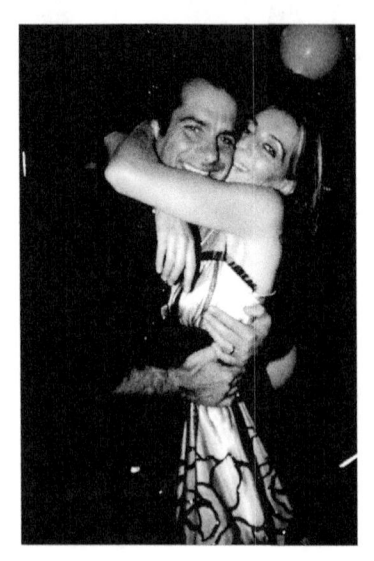

Stefan & Jodi at Sera's Bat Mitzvah party

GALLERY | 55

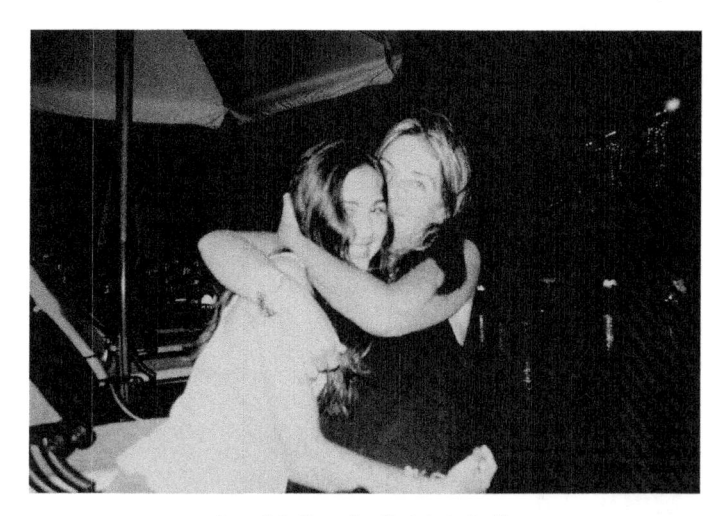

Sera & Jodi on family trip to India

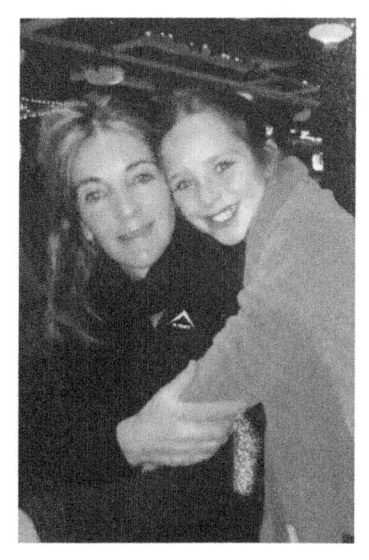

Jodi & Ella, family ski trip in Breckenridge, Colorado

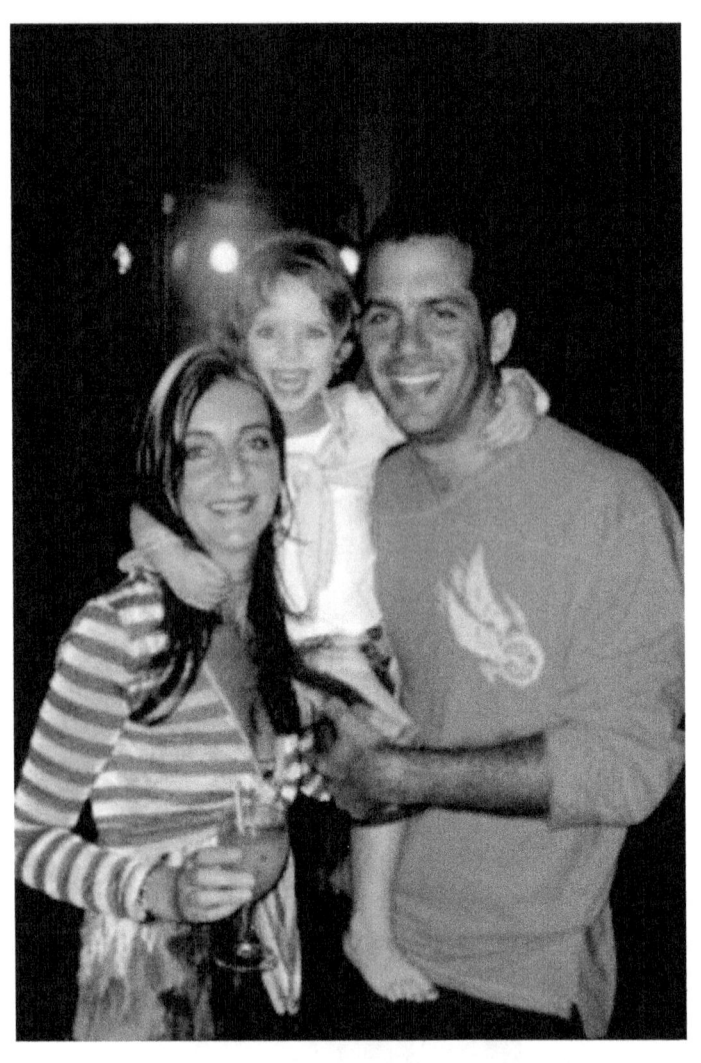

Jodi, Ella & Stefan, at Ella's gratitude party after her heart operation

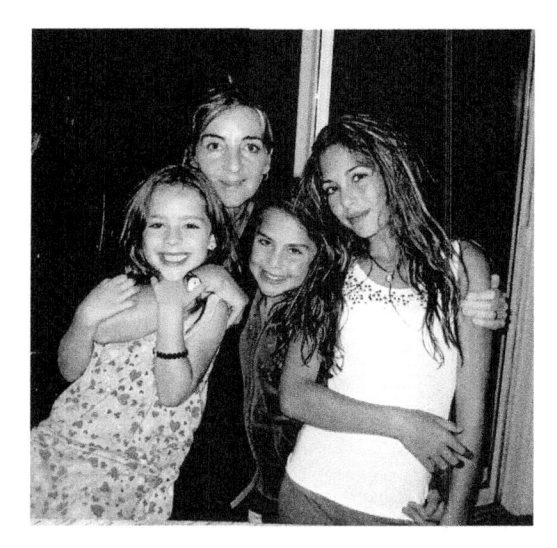

Jodi with her three girls

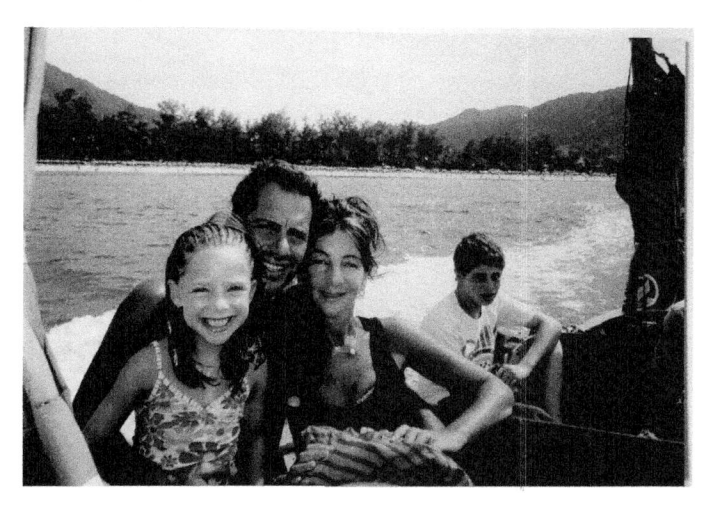

Ella, Stefan & Jodi in Thailand

I found healthy ways not only to feel my feelings
but to express them clearly and to let them go.

The soul exists in the present. The soul is eternal
and understands that life, no matter what
happens to you, is a positive experience.

You have to learn to surrender. Surrendering
means that you nullify your ego and open to
what is—not how you think it should be.

5

EDGING GOD OUT

> "The ego says, 'I shouldn't have to suffer,' and that thought makes you suffer so much more. It is a distortion of the truth, which is always paradoxical. The truth is that you need to say yes to suffering before you can transcend it."
>
> — Eckhart Tolle

A few days after Jodi's diagnosis, friends came over to visit. Within a matter of minutes, I found myself overcome by an intense feeling of claustrophobia—I needed to leave. I decided to go to the gym. It was pitch black as I dived into the outdoor swimming pool. As I swam, I raged, allowing myself to feel all my hurt, anger and fear. With each stroke, I slowly released my emotions. I swam for about half an hour, and then returned to my car. As I sat down in the driver's seat and closed the door, I burst into tears. I don't know how long I sat there in the empty parking lot, but eventually, the tears subsided. I felt as if I had cleansed myself. I started the car and drove back home.

After that evening, exercise became my synagogue. I swam and ran religiously. I would go for a run every Sunday morning, using the time to talk—or rather shout—at God. It would usually go along the lines of, "I can't believe you're doing this to me again, sending me another tumour to have to deal with. It's enough! How can you do this to me? My life is never going to be the same again!" I was seriously pissed off with God, and I allowed myself to express it out loud.

Towards the end of my forty-five-minute run, I could feel the anger subsiding. That's when I would slow down and apologise to God. As I approached our home, I would breathe it all out, literally letting the anger go. When I walked back into the house, I was emotionally strong enough to be there for Jodi and the children. I could be fully present, both as a husband and a father.

My peaceful exterior was not a mask, and my strength was no pretence. I had simply chosen to find healthy ways to feel and release my hurt and anger and frustration. I cried almost every day. It often happened spontaneously, usually while I was driving or running. I did not fight the tears—I chose to welcome them. I would have a good cry for five or ten minutes, and then get on with my day.

Dance, like swimming and running, is a form of release—and emotions must be released. Where do all the feelings go if we don't let them out? Two weeks after my night swim, and even though Jodi was not well enough to accompany me, I decided to go to a friend's fiftieth birthday bash. After a few shots of tequila, I found myself on the dance floor, partying up a storm. I am not sure if anyone at the party was judging me, but I *do* remember wondering if anybody was questioning my having fun while my wife was dying. That night was about being with my mates, celebrating life, and expressing love in a different form.

Something that helped me retain a measure of sanity was choosing to be soul-based over being mind-based. The mind is physical and temporary, whereas the soul is eternal. If I chose to be mind-based, it would mean being ruled by my ego. This would have made me negative, angry and fearful because the mind, by its very nature, lives in the past or the future.

Wayne Dyer, in his book "The Shift: Taking Your Life from Ambition to Meaning", said that when you give in to EGO, you **E**dge **G**od **O**ut—which is precisely what happens when life is all about *you* and what *you* want. A person who is soul-based, on the other hand, sees the bigger picture and understands that life, no matter how it unfolds, is always a positive experience. A soul-based person, knowing that the soul is eternal, exists in the present and gives their life over to the Universe—or God. According to the Torah, when you hand over to God and have faith in the Universe, not only do you trust it implicitly, you allow it to look after you.

But, to be soul-based, you have be prepared to *actually* hand your life over. Most of us cannot or do not want to do that because the pull of the ego is strong. We simultaneously hold mind- and soul-based energies, so we need to recognise when we are aligned with one or the other, and then decide where to place our focus. When I shouted at God and gave over to my emotions, I was aware that I was being mind-based. On days like that, when grief came knocking, I erected a little tent, lit a campfire, and let it in. I allowed myself to surrender into it, to feel the sadness and the sorrow—I just didn't give myself permission to build a house and stay there.

Learning to surrender means nullifying your ego and opening to what *is*—not to how you think things should be. We are tiny specks on this rock floating in the universe, but how often do we refuse to get out of our own way? There must be more at play—it cannot only be about us. God (or the Universe) knows what it is doing and, if it knows what it is doing, perhaps you *don't* know what's truly best for you. When you are open to accepting this, when you can admit that you don't have all the answers, that's when you surrender.

Jodi's body had ended its journey, and her soul was ready to move on. My anger and sadness were for my family, and for me, not for her. I let all my feelings out, and then I let God back in. I accepted what was happening and did not allow the fear, resentment and anger to consume me. I allowed myself to see the beauty of what was unfolding. Being soul-based, I knew that what was happening was not about our physical reality of sickness and death. It was not about a body that is here today and gone tomorrow—it was so much bigger than that.

Ella (16) - We had no choice but to learn

My mom's diagnosis and death changed my

life. It has made me realise that when I don't get an A on a test, or I can't find an outfit to wear, it's not the biggest deal—because there are more important things in life to worry about. If this had never happened, I would have been crying about not having something to wear instead of about how this experience has changed me—for the better. Now, when I cry, I make sure that it is about stuff that matters.

When we understood that what was happening to my mom was serious, it didn't feel real—it felt like a nightmare that I was going to wake up from at any moment. But this was real life, which meant that while we don't know what's going to happen tomorrow, we know, with absolute certainty, that one day we will die. Once you learn to accept this, life begins to carry with it a certain measure of peace.

During those six months, we all changed. We became more conscious, loving and appreciative. We all started getting on. It was beautiful to be a part of it. After dinner, we would all sit around the table, laughing and talking. In the past, we would eat and run—off to our rooms, to our phones, or to watch TV. But we stopped doing that. Instead, we would fight about who would sit next to my mom, and who would help her to eat. Towards the end, when she could no longer brush her teeth or shower herself, I was there, helping her.

Before she got sick, my cell phone was my life. It wasn't long before helping my mom brush her teeth became more important—and more enjoyable—than scrolling through Instagram. My brothers and sisters would stand there while I helped my mom shower and, in those moments, nothing mattered more than the present. I began to understand the meaning of all the signs that my dad had collected and hung around our house. One of them says: "Be happy. This moment is your life".

When I was ten years old, my dad wrote a children's book. In it, he wrote:

To have a God means that you have to accept that there is a power that controls the world—not your ego—and that he is good. The moment we do not accept or surrender to the current situation, we are in the egoist mind state, and we are not practising acceptance, which brings us into the present moment that is soul-based.

I used to grab my mom's cheeks and say, "Mom, you're so cute!" I never said, "Mom, you're so sick!" I wasn't afraid to tell my mom how much I loved her. I will cherish those moments forever. In those last six months of my mom's life, we had fun and laughed more than we had ever laughed as a family. We learned so much.

My mind tells me that I want my mom back, but my soul knows she is at peace. That gives *me* peace. I am grateful for the lessons.

The Universe is a loving place that takes care of me.

If you are open to it, adversity provides an opportunity for presence.

Many of us just want what we want—we don't allow ourselves to be open to what life wants for us. This is a recipe for pain.

Abundance is knowing that the Universe is all-loving, even when it tests us. Everything it gives us is for our ultimate benefit. Our job is simply to say "yes".

POSTSCRIPT

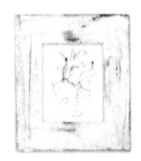

> "Love is a state of being. Your love is not outside, it is deep within you. You can never lose it, and it cannot leave you."
>
> — Eckhart Tolle

We pay a high price when we fall in love—it's a chance we take, and where there is love, one way or another, there is always loss. Jodi and I met in high school, and we got to spend thirty-four glorious years together. Recently, Sera found a speech that Jodi had read at my fortieth. In it, she said that her life had begun when she met me. I cried when I read that. The memories are good. I thank God for them, and I am grateful for the love we had.

Jodi's touch is everywhere in our house—from the well-positioned artwork and the beautiful wallpaper, to the meticulously-framed family photos. Every little thing reminds me of her. Forgetting her is impossible. Each night, I sleep in the bed in which she died. Her final words to us were, "I want you to be happy". That was her directive. As a family, we have chosen to celebrate her life, and I am honouring the love we shared by getting on with my life.

I have a friend whose sister died in childhood. Her mom never got over the death of her child, living her life in the shadow of death. Her other children, who were all very much alive, lived with a terminally-depressed mother whose attention was focused almost entirely on the dead child. Had I died like my friend's mother when Jodi passed away, my children would have lost both parents, and they would not have stood a chance. I chose life because Jodi wanted me to. Because *I* wanted to. Because my children needed me to.

Ella gave me a bookmark that she made with photos of Jodi and me on it. Every night, as I open the book that I am reading, I look at the pictures. It's difficult —a whole lot of emotions come up, but I don't bottle them up. I cry, and then I move on to the next page. I am doing the same with my life. I have children who need to be nurtured and loved by a positive parent who makes them feel the same way. They need to know, and see, that life goes on. Choosing to do this is a call that I made. Some will accuse me of moving on too fast, and that's okay—grief and grieving are deeply personal experiences, and I don't stand in judgement of them.

I am who I am now because of what Jodi taught me and helped me to become. My life is beautiful, and I have her to thank for that. She told me to be happy—it is the most selfless gift she ever gave me. I'm living Jodi's legacy. Honouring her legacy means helping my children to find their happiness too.

I'm alive. The kids are alive. We took the treatments. We took Zanzibar. We took Cape Town. And now we're taking *this* experience. The Universe is a loving place, and it is taking care of us.

Being happy after Jodi left us wasn't something that happened overnight—it was a process. This experience forced each of us to enjoy *the now* because the present only comes around once. As I found my new sense of normal, I slowly found more minutes in the day to be present. These days, I experience *hours* of presence. My life is a continuous journey towards living in the now.

If you are open to it, adversity provides an opportunity for presence. When you are open to life teaching you, then you will be a little more prepared for what it throws your way. I lost my father and went on a journey of trying to understand how the Universe works, and the Universe provided me with ample opportunities to learn about it and connect with it.

Many of us just want what we want—we don't allow ourselves to be open to what life wants for us. This is a recipe for pain. I have been extremely blessed in that I have never wanted for anything materially. My father left us well-off, and I have also made plenty of money of my own through various business endeavours. Although I have an abundance mentality, I have come to realise that abundance is not just about money. Many people have plenty of money, but they have a scarcity mentality. Their fear of losing it all consumes them, and they walk around, filled with anxiety. A true abundance mentality is knowing, and trusting, that the Universe is all-loving, even when it tests us. We need to remember that what it gives us is for our ultimate benefit. All we have to do is say, "Yes".

While in the sauna at gym recently, I was chatting to a doctor. He asked me if the treatment, which, in the end, was unable to save Jodi's life, was worth it—and would I recommend it. Almost two years after Jodi's death, and with the added benefit of hindsight, I told him that yes, it was worth it. I explained how our time spent with Jodi was quality time. I told him how the experience was our training ground to learn how *not* to be gripped by fear. Allowing our thoughts to run away with us, no matter how uncertain the future looked, was a great, big no-no. We were willing to embrace the experience, no matter the outcome. Overthinking and stressing about how things were going to turn out would not have served us—the experience of watching a loved one die is difficult enough. We had to make peace with our choices and use them to make us better, not bitter. What other choice do we have in the face of unavoidable suffering?

Jodi loved the book by Terry Hayes called "I am Pilgrim". It is an escapist adventure story, nothing deep or meaningful. In the book, the author quotes Robert Louis Stevenson, who said:

> "Sooner or later, we all sit down
> to a banquet of consequences."

Life is all about choices. We are free to choose, but we are not free from the consequences of those choices. As you go forth in life, make healthy choices. Ensure that the banquet you sit down to is a festive one.

READING LIST

Books mentioned

Brozin, Stefan (2012). TREE. United States: Eloquent Books

Dyer, Wayne (2019). The Shift: Taking Your Life from Ambition to Meaning. Carlsbad, CA: Hay House

Frankl, V. E. (1984). Man's Search for Meaning: An Introduction to Logotherapy. New York: Simon & Schuster

Hayes, Terry (2014). I am Pilgrim. Washington: Atria Books

Singer, M. A. (2007). The Untethered Soul: The Journey Beyond Yourself. Oakland, CA: New Harbinger Publications

Tolle, Eckhart (2004). The Power of Now: A Guide to Spiritual Enlightenment. Vancouver: Namaste Publishing

Stef's Recommended Reading

Arush, Shalom and Brody, Lazer (2007). The Garden

of Emunah: A Practical Guide to Life. New York: Feldheim Publishers

Parthasarathy, A. (2004). The Eternities - Vedanta Treatise. Mumbai, India: Vedanta Life Institute

Singer, M. A. (2015). The Surrender Experiment: My Journey into Life's Perfection. New York: Random House USA Inc.

Tolle, Eckhart (2001). Practicing the Power of Now: Meditations, Exercises, and Core Teachings for Living the Liberated Life. Novato, CA: New World Library

Tolle, Eckhart (2009). A New Earth: Awakening to Your Life's Purpose. London: Penguin Books Ltd

NOTES

2. LITTLE ME; BIG ME

1. Tolle, Eckhart (1997). The Power of Now: A Guide to Spiritual Enlightenment. Vancouver: Namaste Publishing
2. Singer, M. A. (2007). The Untethered Soul: The Journey Beyond Yourself. Oakland, CA: New Harbinger Publications

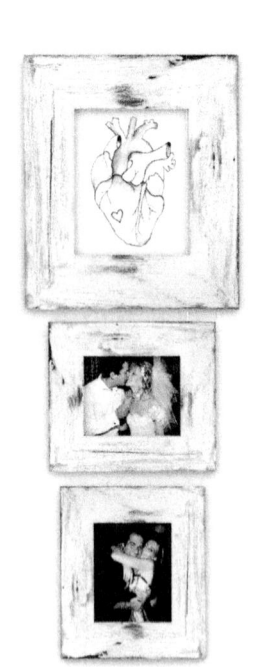

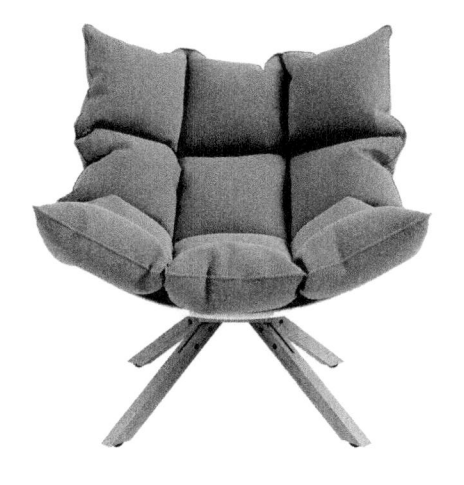

Printed in Great Britain
by Amazon